PENGUIN BOOKS

GIVING COMFORT

Born and raised in Michigan, and a graduate of
the University of Michigan, Linda Breiner Milstein worked as a preschool teacher and infant
development researcher in Ann Arbor before
moving to New York City to attend the Wurz-
weiler School of Social Work at Yeshiva University. While working in oncology at Mount
Sinai Hospital she also pursued training in child
psychotherapy, later working as a child therapist. After the birth of her second child she
turned her attention to writing children's books
and inventing toys. This is her first adult non-
fiction book. She lives in Westchester with her
husband, son and daughter.

GIVING COMFORT

What You Can Do When Someone You Love Is Ill

LINDA BREINER MILSTEIN

Penguin Books

PENGUIN BOOKS
Published by the Penguin Group
Penguin Books USA Inc., 375 Hudson Street,
New York, New York 10014, U.S.A.
Penguin Books Ltd, 27 Wrights Lane,
London W8 5TZ, England
Penguin Books Australia Ltd, Ringwood,
Victoria, Australia
Penguin Books Canada Ltd, 10 Alcorn Avenue,
Toronto, Ontario, Canada M4V 3B2
Penguin Books (N.Z.) Ltd, 182–190 Wairau Road,
Auckland 10, New Zealand

Penguin Books Ltd, Registered Offices:
Harmondsworth, Middlesex, England

First published in Penguin Books 1994

1 3 5 7 9 10 8 6 4 2

LIBRARY OF CONGRESS CATALOGING IN PUBLICATION DATA
Milstein, Linda Breiner.
Giving comfort : What You Can Do When Someone You Love Is Ill /
Linda Breiner Milstein.
p. cm.
Includes bibliographical references.
ISBN 0 14 02.3538 8
1. Hospital care—Psychological aspects. 2. Hospital patients—
Psychology. 3. Caregivers. I. Title.
RA965.3.M55 1994
610.73—dc20   93-32169

Printed in the United States of America
Set in Goudy Old Style
Designed by Katy Riegel

To Sam,

whose love made this possible,

with all my love

Preface

❖ While my cousin Paula was in the final stages of breast cancer, I told a friend about my visits to the hospital. She was surprised by what I did. Not that anything was so unusual, it was because everything was so simple. But like the perfect line thought of too late, or not at all, it can be hard to know what to say or do when you are in the throes of emotion that a gravely ill loved one inspires. Months after Paula's death, I wrote down a few of my better ideas for extending comfort and gave the list to a friend. Out of that sharing grew the idea for this book.

Writing these suggestions and meditations down has been difficult and rewarding in equal measure. I had to relive, painfully, my farewell to Paula—indeed, our whole relationship over the years. I also had the opportunity to turn my grief into something positive. Paula would have liked that. Like myself, she was a social worker. My model and mentor, she fervently believed in enabling people to help themselves. She made a fine art of appreciating each person and each moment's uniqueness, and always made the best of whatever came along. Her gift to me was to embody and demonstrate that spirit. I have tried to return that gift to her by capturing it in these pages.

I cannot take credit for creating all these ideas on my own. Some were the result of kindnesses extended to me by others. Some were suggested by the friends who so generously read this manuscript, allowing their old scars to be reopened. Much of the material for this book came out of my work at Mount Sinai Hospital in New York. As the social worker in The Out-Patient Neoplastic and Hematology-Chemotherapy Clinics as well as The Breast Service, I saw hundreds of people and their families, following them on their odyssey through clinic and hospital. My background in early childhood education and infant development put me in an excellent position to work with people experiencing serious illness. The areas of early development and illness share a major concern with issues of attachment and loss, autonomy and dependence, styles of coping with anxiety and aggression, and the boundaries of Self and Other. The experiences packed into the two years I spent in oncology resonated with these themes and strongly influenced my subsequent work as a child therapist.

Working within the specialized, interdisciplinary medical team at Mount Sinai, seeing the same patients and their loved ones on a weekly, even a daily, basis in health, in illness, in treatment, in death, and in bereavement over the course of two years—this was a rare privilege. The physicians with whom I worked were as compassionate as they were dedicated. The support staff always gave something extra for our patients. Most especially, it was the oncology nurses who inspired and challenged me every day. Their wisdom is heavily laced into these pages and I am forever in their debt for all I learned standing by their side. But it is mainly to our patients and their friends and families that I most deeply bow. I received far more than I could ever give back. I am truly humbled by their courage and ingenuity.

As I wrote this book, their faces rose before my eyes. In my imagination I had the chance to do things over again, better. I forgave myself for all I did not know at crucial moments, comforted by all I had since learned and was now in a position to pass on. As wonderful as that feeling is, it was also enervating to relive, within a relatively short period, the hundred or so deaths I was a party to during my tenure at Mount Sinai. It is with a satisfied, almost joyful sigh that I have completed this book, part guide, part memoir.

Acknowledgments

❖ I wish to acknowledge my debt, with heartfelt thanks, to Miriam Rubin, Elizabeth Ehrlich, and Hannah Parnes, whose friendship, encouragement, and sound suggestions gave this book its start, and whose lives have taught me more than they can know. I gratefully thank Elisa Petrini, whose literary guidance, professional advice, and personal encouragement were crucial in developing this idea into a tangible reality. I thank Karen Mesberg, my friend and neighbor, who gladly read this, and everything else I have ever written, over and over, always with care and candor, no matter how busy she was. A thank you to my father, Sander Breiner, my aunt and uncle Lynn and Allan Oboler, and my friend Jean Parvin Bordewich for their helpful comments and their confidence in this project. To my mother, Beatrice Breiner, a special thank you. It was her untiring efforts on the computer at a crucial stage that kept the project on schedule, and it was her untiring generosity all my life that fed the wellsprings of this book. I have happily had the great good fortune of having Susan Cohen as my agent and Mindy Werner as my editor; two more perceptive, decisive, energetic women I cannot imagine. I wish to extend a huge thank you to them and the entire staff at Penguin for believing in this book with such enthusiasm. My thanks would be incomplete without acknowledging the importance of my loving memories of Paula Schwartz and Elaine Heumann. They taught and inspired me in their lives, and in their dying. And I thank the honored memories of two people whom I never knew, but whose legacies have helped shape this writing, Noach Milstein and Anat Parzenchevski. I hope my small knowledge of their lives, distilled into this book, has added some meaning to their untimely passing. And especially to my husband, Sam, and my children, Noah and Zena, the most enormous thank you for putting up with much, for making room in their lives, for their love, encouragement, patience, good humor, and pride.

Contents

Introduction

❖ You're looking for something, but you're not sure what. It might help to escape into a book, but it's hard for you to concentrate lately. Someone you love is ill, perhaps very ill, and you want to know what you can do. You want answers, but you're not sure of the questions, or whom to ask. You want information, but you don't know where to look. You wish there was something you could do, really *do* for your loved one. Meanwhile, you want to know what to do with your hands, your feelings, your thoughts, your time. You want to help, but how? You yourself need help to figure out this strange world of illness, but you don't know where to begin.

I think I have known you, or someone like you. You've visited your loved one who is ill. You have said all the right things, you think, but something is missing. Or maybe there is something more you can do. But your loved one doesn't ask and nobody else around seems to have any ideas. You feel awkward. You are new at this, this sick business, and you don't think you're very good at it. Or perhaps you are, and always have been, uncomfortable around illness. You are a little frightened by this new experience, and that embarrasses you. Or perhaps you are consumed with your feelings for your loved one and can't seem to think straight, much less creatively, within these emotions.

These are all natural reactions to an unhappy situation. Knowing that may reassure you, but it won't help you much. There are, however, things that you can do to live with your loved one's illness better. This is a book for you. This is a book about your needs: your need to help, understand, be there, do something, and comfort your loved one. This is a book about how to give, how to make your efforts count for you, and for your loved one. This is a book about how to spend time effectively, how to live with the situation.

And what is that situation? It is one of great difficulty. You care about someone and that person is sick or hurt. Perhaps it is an accident or an illness from which your loved one will fully recover. Or maybe your loved one has a chronic condition which, though debilitating, can be lived with for a long time to come. Perhaps your loved one's condition is deteriorating and you face new handicaps, new restrictions, more treatment. Perhaps your loved one has a severe illness and is engaged in an intense struggle to "beat the thing." Or maybe you are adjusting to a new diagnosis or a medical condition that suddenly, abruptly struck your loved one out of the blue, turning your world upside down.

You might be facing the final stages of your loved one's terminal illness. Perhaps your loved one is actively dying at this moment. Whatever the particular medical condition is that brings you to consider the subject of illness, however unique your circumstances, you are united with thousands of others who, like you, love someone who is now hurt, ill, or in some way incapacitated. And whatever your particular relationship is to your loved one, you want to reach out and give comfort.

And who are you? You are the spouse, or the child, or a close family member, a distant relative, an ex-boyfriend, a fiancé. You are an old friend with a long history. You are a neighbor, a lover, a colleague, a family friend since childhood. You are your loved one's very dearest, closest friend. You are only an acquaintance, but you truly care.

This book is written for you. It is the companion you can turn to for advice when you're uncertain. Not all of what this book has to say will apply to you. But whoever you are, whatever the situation you face with your loved one, the suggestions that you need in order to learn how to give comfort can be found here. For the most part I have alternated the gender of the patient from chapter to chapter. That is because the suggestions and descriptions are valid for both sexes. Skim through the pages, pick and choose the ideas that apply to you and your circumstances. Gauge what suits you, your personality, the personality of your loved one, his needs and your relationship. You will be able to tell what is right for you. Take whatever you can use, and ignore the rest.

Much of what I've written seems to assume hospitalization and a life-threatening illness. I purposefully chose to speak in the extremes of ordinary health care and experience to be sure to include everyone. Situations where the illness is being treated at home or is less severe, mild, temporary, or reversible will all benefit from most of the suggestions set forth here. The vast majority of all patients are cared for at home for most of their convalescence. Indeed, the primary goal of hospitalization is to return the patient home for further care and eventual cure in the home setting. The unsung heroes of health care are and always were the friends and family who care for and comfort their loved ones at home. This book is written with you in mind. The ideas in it are meant to travel well between home and hospital, between sprained ankles and major surgeries.

You'll find too that certain important ideas and suggestions are repeated in several places. I want you to be able to easily find the information that will be most useful to you without having to cull through every word to get at it.

I have tried to describe what to look and listen for, what issues may be important, what approach you might take in response, how, even, to frame your response. At the same time I have kept firmly in mind that whatever action you, the reader, might take, your words are and should be your own, as unique and personal as your relationship to your loved one. I have therefore tried to give you some hints and tools that can help you interpret what is going on before you, without dictating exactly which words to say. It is my hope that you will be better equipped to make your best, most genuine response if you understand better what might be going on within your loved one and the type of things you might do to give comfort.

Although need, confusion, even frustration may have guided you to this book, although sadness surely lingers at the edges of these thoughts, it is not the emotion that most empowers these words. Behind them stands great love and affection. That is why I frequently refer to the focus of your attention as "your loved one" rather than "the patient." And that is why you have turned to these pages in the first place. Let that feeling of affection be your guide in choosing how you comfort your loved one. After all, the only criterion for giving comfort is to care. Help your loved one cope with illness and, if it comes to that, face dying. Comfort your loved one. Be involved. It is a journey worth taking.

PART ONE

Ways of Being

1

Give Friendly Comfort

❖ Your loved one is in the hospital. What does that mean? She is away from home, alone and uncomfortable. No matter how advanced the hospital is, nor how great the care given, it is still a place built to help people in physical need. It is bustling and intrusive and unfamiliar and utilitarian. And your loved one is in it. And she is ill, and requires expert medical attention.

But you have something quite special and wonderful that your loved one wants. It is something no hospital can provide but every ill person desperately needs. The best, the very best thing you have to offer is your companionship. Your presence alone is an enormous help. Here are some ways you can share it with your loved one.

❖ *1.* Show you care by simply being there. Without bringing anything to give, without knowing anything

to do, without having anything to say, you—your presence—will make your loved one feel better.

❖ 2. Make short, frequent visits that will not wear you or
your loved one out. Don't stay so long that you find it too
hard to return another day. Then the person you love can
be comforted by knowing you will return, even if only for a
brief time.

❖ 3. If she is tired and weak, she may simply like to hear
your voice, in person or over the phone, even if she doesn't
feel like talking. Tell your loved one about your day's events,
a joke, a news item, or the weather for a few minutes without making any demands on her sociability.

❖ 4. Help your loved one keep friendships going. Urge
her to keep in touch with the people in her life. Urge
friends, family, and co-workers to respond and reach out.
With her consent, offer to be the liaison that keeps the
communication going with others. Set up a telephone tree
to relay information about her. You can volunteer to be the
collection center for written and verbal messages.

❖ 5. Be a friendly listener. Be that special person who is
willing to talk about anything, happy or sad, important or
trivial, without censure.

❖ 6. Be an honest friend. Answer her questions openly
and truthfully. If you don't know the answer, do not be

afraid to say so. But do not shy away from discussing certain topics or using certain words related to your loved one's illness. You may be afraid to upset her. But there is nothing you can say about your loved one's illness that she hasn't already thought of in private. There is nothing so frightening as being alone with troubling thoughts and thinking there is no one you can really talk to.

2

Give Hopeful Comfort

❖ There is something new in your loved one's life, and it is not welcome. He is ill and that fact affects everything. Illness is always an intrusion upon the normal pace and flavor of life. No matter how many symptoms may have helped your loved one anticipate the diagnosis, it will still feel abrupt. The experience of disruption is all the more harsh if your loved one is suffering the ill effects of an accident. But even if he has long lived with a chronic condition that has only recently deteriorated or presented complications, those changes from life's familiar pattern may be as disheartening as an initial diagnosis, even though the changes might have been anticipated.

Your loved one did not want to be introduced into this world of illness. Yet here he is, forced to play out his role as patient as best he can. He may be bewildered, anxious, angry, or depressed over his situation. Chances are he will feel these and many other emotions, repeatedly, over the course of his illness. It will be a great challenge for him to maintain hope while he simultaneously allows himself to explore and express the other thoughts and feelings that are part of this experience.

You want him to have hope, to go forth with a fighting spirit. But you too may be subject to the same onslaught of concerns and feelings as your loved one. You will need to muster your sources of hope as surely as your loved one will. And what exactly is hope? Hope is anything that allows the individual to carry on in the most advantageous way possible. It does not obstruct. Hope is constructive. Hope can be a potent enhancement to healing, wellness, and the treatment of illness. Its content cannot be prescribed. It will differ for each person. Hope may alter its shape over time, adapting to the changing circumstances of illness. But as long as it doesn't mislead in a harmful manner, it can comfort your loved one while being of immense benefit to his treatment prospects.

Hope can be a powerful agent in healing. The medical staff certainly does not want to destroy hope at any juncture. Hope and medicine are allies in this struggle. But hope does not always grow comfortably next to realism. Helping your loved one find a way for his hope and the realistic needs of his medical condition to coexist will be a great boon to his health and well-being. He has a big job ahead of him. He must get as well as he can, cope as effectively as he can, and remain as whole as he can. You can bring him comfort by helping him feel hopeful should he become overwhelmed by these difficult tasks.

Hope and faith are intertwined: faith in doctors; in a higher power; in science; in love; in one's own strength, character, and abilities; in another person's affection and loyalty. Letting your loved one know that he can and should have faith in the things that are important to him can go a long way toward supporting or restoring his important sense of hopefulness.

❖ 7. Help him find hope in his faith, spiritual or personal.

❖ 8. Help him find hope in science, in the belief that people are trying to find the answers he seeks, that someone has or will soon have the medical knowledge and assistance that he needs.

❖ 9. Help him have faith in time—in the adjustments, mending, growth, and answers that it can bring.

❖ 10. Help him have faith in himself—in his ability to aid in his own healing through effort, attention, love, stress reduction, affection, and confidence.

❖ 11. Don't accept defeat. Demand your loved one not give up without a fight.

❖ *12.* Create hope by helping him explore his options. Review the plans presented by his doctors. Help him seek additional opinions, locate information, and explore the range of treatment options and other resources. (See chapter 31, "Resources for Comfort.")

❖ *13.* Find inspiration, encouragement, and borrowed strength in the success stories of other patients' struggles. The knowledge that he is not unique in his concerns, that others have met similar challenges and have managed with the same burdens can instill a sense of hope as he faces what must otherwise feel like a lone battle.

❖ *14.* Build hope within your loved one. Identify and celebrate his successes at overcoming previous obstacles in life. Nurture his inner strength and trust in his own abilities to meet this new challenge of illness.

❖ *15.* Be supportive of the trust he places in his medical team, especially his physician. Having trust in his medical care is closely related to his sense of security and therefore his sense of hopefulness.

❖ *16.* Build hope by coping. Helping your loved one cope with the immediate problems of logistics and concerns over initial diagnosis and treatment can give him concrete evidence that the issues illness presents can be rationally dealt with one at a time. Helping him explore and plan for future needs demonstrates your hope in him, and in the future you will share. It also demonstrates that you have not given up on him in despair, fear, or disinterest, but do indeed have hope for the future.

3

Give
Accepting Comfort

❖ Illness has involved your loved one in a drama not of her choosing, that she cannot walk away from. Our inability as human beings to protect ourselves fully against illness and accidents, or to control our bodies' reactions to such things, is a potent example of our own ultimate powerlessness. Your loved one may well be struggling with these issues as she tries to cope with her illness. She may experience extremes of emotion that you do not ordinarily associate with her. You may find the expression of these feelings, including depression, rage, fearfulness, confusion, so unfamiliar, or at times unfounded, as to make you wonder if your loved one has become a different person.

Your loved one has indeed changed. She has had to confront the fallibility, the imperfection, the very breakdown of her body. Such a profound awareness has different meanings for all of us. But it is never a negligible event. Your loved

one may feel fear for what is to come, regret or disappoint-
ment for what is past, confusion, frustration, or hurt over
what is occurring. There may be an attempt to assign blame
for her present circumstances, anger or guilt accompanying
such thoughts. There may be words of grief, or jealousy, or
anger over what was left undone, unfinished, and is now
difficult or unattainable. Any perceived time pressure may
condense and amplify these emotions, especially if your
loved one is missing out on an important occasion due to
illness or feels she is facing permanent disability or death.

Sometimes your loved one may direct these sentiments
toward the doctors and nurses simply because they are the
ones who are most involved in her daily existence. Or the
hospital staff may become a target of your loved one's distress because they have not fulfilled the entirely natural
hope of receiving a quick and complete cure and being res-
cued from the illness. Sometimes her upset (and upsetting)
feelings may be directed toward you. This may seem unfair.
But it can be much too threatening for your loved one to
show anger, even deserved anger, toward the hospital staff
on whom she is now so dependent for basic needs. You may
become the undeserved recipient of these feelings precisely
because you are the very person who loves, the safe person
to complain to, or about, in a world that has spun wildly
out of her control.

Angry complaints about unimportant issues, or unrealistic expectations, often express hopes and fears on subjects
that may otherwise be too painful to broach. You can be
supportive of your loved one's struggle to make sense of all

these difficult, conflicting, and challenging emotions. It is not your arguments or your agreement that she ultimately needs. It is your acceptance of all she is, and despite all of what she may say, that counts and is most comforting.

❖ **17.** Listen unreservedly to your loved one's reports of her physical and medical changes and routines. Even the least hypochondriacal person will shift greater attention onto the minute changes in her physical status as her world shrinks to the dimensions of a single room, or even a bed.

❖ **18.** Listen tolerantly to your loved one's anger at old wounds, new hurts, life, the current situation. Listen uncritically to complaints, large and small, real and imagined.

❖ **19.** Listen bravely to your loved one's fears, worries, and uncertainties. Help her sort them out and face these concerns together. There is nothing so lonely as thinking you exist without having any shared feeling of understanding with another human being. You cannot truly travel with your loved one on the road into this illness. But you can accompany this special person in facing her secret concerns.

❖ **20.** Listen compassionately to your loved one's treatment plans (or plans to refuse treatment). Help her examine whether these are impulsive choices or actions that are consistent with long-held beliefs. Help her be true to herself and make the best possible choice. Accept who your loved is and what she does.

❖ 2 1. Praise your loved one for all the good things in her life. Appreciate the positive: her good qualities, friendships, and happy experiences. Articulate these things for her. Remind and review with her all she has accomplished, overcome, achieved, and all those who care about her.

❖ 2 2. Forgive your loved one for past grievances. Try to put current grievances into context. Are they related to the illness or part of a longer history? Do they really matter at all or can they be overlooked? Focus on what is important in your relationship and ignore the rest. Be generous. Be accepting.

4

Give
Inspirational Comfort

❖ After becoming ill, your loved one may seem suddenly to develop new ideas or deeper feelings about faith, life, and death. Religion may suddenly hold a greater interest for your loved one than ever before in your experience. This is a natural phenomenon. Many people do not solidify or even explore their views on faith and spirituality until they are faced with the crisis of their own mortality. For others, the same experience can undermine their equilibrium, throwing long-held beliefs (and disbeliefs) into question. Following your loved one's cues, you can help him make good use of this transitional period. It can be a time of philosophical growth and clarification. You can assist and support your loved one in exploring the traditional and nontraditional spiritual sources of comfort, strength, and inspiration that appeal to him.

If you are unsure or unfamiliar with your loved one's religious beliefs, ask him. If he has no religious affiliation at this time, or has expressed no special interest in this area, but has a background connected with a particular tradition, ask about it. Demonstrate that you are open to exploring this potential source of comfort with him. Ask what feels right to him. But above all, ask.

❖ 23. Approve. Without judging, allow your loved one to express these thoughts and feelings. Without imposing answers, offer assistance in seeking them.

❖ 24. Pray. If there are particular prayers that are meaningful to your loved one, pray together.

❖ 25. Cherish. If there are religious or personal objects of special significance to your loved one, bring them to the hospital to be used and cherished.

❖ 26. Read. If there is liturgy, poetry, or literature that is especially meaningful for your loved one, read it aloud.

❖ 27. Visit. If there is a clergy member whose words would be helpful to your loved one, arrange for that person to visit.

❖ **28.** Notify. Keep congregation members informed so they can call, write, pray, and think about your loved one.

❖ **29.** Listen. Play tapes of favorite liturgical music.

❖ **30.** Sing. If there is music that is especially meaningful for your loved one, share the intimacy of your voice.

5

Give
Understanding Comfort

❖ Your loved one will have lots of questions and concerns, large and small, about what is happening to and around her. It may be difficult to put some of these thoughts into words, out of anxiety or just plain fatigue. Perhaps she is feeling too exhausted to truly hear and take in the information that is being offered. Perhaps events are unfolding too quickly to keep up with, and she has not had enough time to formulate her questions. Understanding what is going on around her will be one of the greatest sources of comfort you can give your loved one. Ensuring that the necessary clear communication takes place will be a significant contribution toward her comfort.

Clear communication does not mean a perfectly worded statement. It can be difficult the first time around for your loved one to really hear, retain, and appreciate much of what is being said regarding her illness, treatment options, and the hospital routines. The whole situation is often so stressful that pieces of the official explanations can get turned around, glossed over, misunderstood, emphasized differently over time, and just plain forgotten. Questions your loved one wants answered can easily get overlooked in the rushed moments when the nurse or physician is present and the conversation is focused on a subject different from your loved one's original concern. Important details get lost amid all the new information she must cope with. Clear communication means making everything well understood to all the participants. In order for communication to be clear when the subject matter is so stressful, information should be repeated and discussed, more than once.

Clear communication and candor go together. There can be no true understanding if the discussion is built on euphemisms, evasion, half-truths, or platitudes. But just what is candor? Candor is truthfulness. But like clear communication, candor is never brutal, even in the service of telling the truth. Candor implies sensitivity to the needs and emotional capacity of the listener. When good, clear communication has been established and all parties are speaking with candor, then your loved one should be able to comprehend and use the information presented. That is the goal and the ideal. Achieving it will take effort. Your assistance can make the difference for her between the comfort of having understood what is going on and the anxiety of living with unnecessary ambiguity and uncertainty. It is not up to you, of course, to present any medically related information to your loved one. That is the job of the physician. The doctor will discuss diagnosis, prognosis, treatment options, side effects, and introduce the vocabulary needed to discuss your loved one's health.

Some of the most important and comforting information being sought may not seem momentous to you. Perhaps your loved one is concerned about gastric distress and is fearful of being helpless with her discomfort during the night when the doctor is not around. It can be a great source of comfort to ask about what provisions have been made for this possibility and find out that medical orders for a helpful prescription have been left in the chart, should it occur. Such information can put the patient's mind at ease. Whatever the subject, when you help your loved one formulate her questions and obtain the needed answers, you are helping replace anxieties with understanding and thereby giving her a form of comfort that will outlast any flower arrangement.

❖ 31. Urge your loved one to write down questions as they occur so they can be answered later when the opportunity arises.

❖ 32. Urge your loved one to write down the answers to her questions or use a tape recorder. Offer to assist with this task. A taped or written record can be reviewed to remind her later exactly what was said.

❖ *33.* Urge your loved one to write down the pertinent medical terms employed by the doctor. Ask about the meanings if they are unclear. Being specific and accurate will help avoid confusion.

❖ *34.* Use the same vocabulary the physician and your loved one employ. If she is using a term, avoid substituting euphemisms that obscure. Using the same accurate vocabulary opens up the opportunity for your loved one to speak frankly with you about important personal matters.

❖ *35.* Urge your loved one to review the information she wrote down at a later time. More questions may arise in the interim. Remind her that asking the same questions over again is a natural and important part of the process of understanding.

❖ *36.* Urge your loved one to ask systematically about medication and procedures. Urge her to get an explanation in detail so she will know what to anticipate.

❖ *37.* Ask your loved one what problems she is experiencing. Ask what her concerns and expectations are. Help her articulate her curiosity and anxiety so they can be formulated into questions to be asked later.

❖ *38.* Ask your loved one if she feels comfortable and what might be done to make her more comfortable. Help her convey this information to those who can help.

❖ *39.* Help your loved one have good communication with her friends and family. Offer to write down and/or convey personal messages, requests, and questions.

❖ *40.* Offer to set up a telephone tree among family and friends so the people in your loved one's world can be kept informed.

❖ *41.* As an interested party, communicate your concerns and observations to the physician or nurse on duty. While they are ethically bound not to discuss anything without the patient's express permission, your input may enhance their communication with the patient.

❖ *42.* When your loved one is at home, it is especially important to record instructions and explanations. In the hospital she is constantly monitored as part of the medical care system. In order to provide the best possible care while at home, it is even more important to convey her questions and describe any changes promptly and accurately to the visiting nurse and physician.

PART TWO

---

*Things
You Can Bring*

6

Bring Comfort Food

❖ You want to do something for your loved one, but you don't know what. You know you want to make him feel better, to cheer him up, to distract him from thoughts of illness, to give him your love, some enjoyment, to take care of him. What can you possibly do, you wonder. So you think of what you can bring to your loved one. Food, maybe. Food has always given pleasure in the past. You've celebrated happy events over good meals and soothed hurts with special treats. Food is a natural choice and a good place to start.

But before you pack a basket of goodies, ask your loved one what he might enjoy. Old assumptions may not hold true. Your loved one may not want, or be able, to eat regular food because of the effects of the medical treatment or the disease process itself. For the same reasons, compounded by the dry hospital air, your loved one may be experiencing a period of extremely tender, sensitive mouth and gums, or a dry mouth. Because of illness or treatment, he may be having difficulty holding food down or having trouble with digestion or elimination. Side effects of treatment or the illness can also create food or odor aversions, odd cravings, or render once-favorite foods distasteful. He may be too tired to eat in a conventional manner (sitting upright with a knife and fork), or no longer enjoy former favorites that require extensive cutting or chewing. And the three-meals-a-day food service of a large institutional kitchen may not suit his diminished appetite, which requires smaller, more frequent servings.

Don't be surprised if the entire subject of food and related areas—appetite, meal delivery, digestion—evokes stronger than expected reactions in your loved one. What goes in and out of one's body in the hospital is a major focus and duly noted by the medical staff, drawing your loved one's attention to food and its effects with a greater than usual intensity.

More important, your loved one's feelings on other subjects can easily get displaced onto the food provided. It is so much easier to complain about one's diet than one's health. Food is a safe and convenient focus for the anger and distress your loved one will experience at times. It feels less risky to reject food than to complain about the doctor or the medical treatment.

It is also likely to be the first time since infancy that your loved one is completely dependent on others for sustenance. This lack of control over such a basic need and pleasure as eating can bring out a host of emotions including anger and depression. Also, the disruption of lifelong eating patterns may be emotionally charged itself, taking on great symbolism for the patient and requiring your utmost sensitivity.

Bearing all this in mind, you can still bring things that will probably please and appeal. But always remember to check with your loved one about his desires and with the appropriate medical staff about any food restrictions before following any suggestions here or elsewhere in this book.

❖ *43.* Ask the clerk at the nursing station about kitchen resources. There should be a room on the floor with a microwave oven, ice machine, and refrigerator or freezer available for patient and visitor use. It may also be possible to rent a small fridge for the room.

❖ *44.* In a wide-mouthed Thermos, bring homemade chicken noodle soup, or any other mild, broth-based favorite containing small pieces of well-cooked, and easily chewable and digestible food. This can be kept bedside and consumed throughout the day, a few mouthfuls at a time.

❖ *45.* Bring small amounts of fruit-flavored sherbet. If refrigeration is a problem, transfer some to a shallow wide-mouthed Thermos so it can be eaten slowly over the course of several hours.

❖ *46.* Bring a supply of chilled nutritional supplements such as shakes or puddings by Ensure or Sustical (available from pharmacies, surgical supply stores, or the hospital dietitian). Chocolate- and coffee-flavored products are popular.

❖ 47. Bring some lunchbox-sized snack packs of puddings, applesauce, fruit cocktail. They are small, require no chewing, no refrigeration, and tend to be low in acid, good for sensitive mouths and stomachs.

❖ 48. Bring a container of assorted small hard candies to be kept bedside. They provide a pleasant taste and temporarily relieve dry mouth.

❖ 49. Bring some dried fruit for munching at all hours.

❖ 50. Bring clementines, seedless grapes, cubed melon, or other juicy, nonacidic fruit for snacking.

❖ 51. Bring a package of light cookies or crackers that are low in too-rich-to-digest butterfat, such as saltines, rice crackers, and cholesterol-free snack products.

❖ 52. Bring an assortment of juices not available in the hospital. Choose the single-serving snack packs of boxes or cans.

❖ 53. Bring an emergency bottle of seltzer or water with a twist top to be kept bedside in case other liquids run out during the night and attendants are not immediately available.

❖ *54.* Bring a Thermos or pitcher of ice water to be kept bedside. You can replenish the ice from an ice machine on the floor. Ask for directions at the nursing station.

❖ *55.* Bring a Thermos of hot water and a choice of herbal teas to be kept bedside. (Some stores carry a push-button, easy-to-pour carafe that looks like a pitcher but retains heat and does not spill.)

❖ *56.* Bring a covered plastic car mug or child's cup for sipping in bed.

❖ *57.* Bring a supply of disposable spoons, cups, and flexible straws.

7

Bring Body Comfort

❖ Try to imagine the experience of immobilization. Now add to that the side effects of illness and treatment, and the physical restrictions and intrusions imposed by hospital routine. Any and all of the usual self-care habits that your loved one takes for granted, such as grooming, dressing, or washing, may be impossible to perform without some kind of assistance. She may need someone to accompany her to the toilet if she is weak and in danger of falling. If she is not able to get out of bed and is using a bedpan, she will need the assistance of others to put it in place and remove it. These and other such experiences of dependence, of having to ask—and wait—for help to accomplish even the smallest, most ordinary of actions, from bathing to straightening the blankets, will almost certainly affect your loved one.

Anticipating needs requires empathy and imagination on your part. It is a balancing act to know just how much or how little to do for your loved one, and when. You must weigh the effects of dependence and independence at a given moment, sometimes encouraging effort, sometimes offering help. You will need to be flexible. Whatever you assess the situation to be, as your loved one's condition changes, so too will these most personal of needs.

Often, the medical staff can provide special aids for the patient's comfort from a hospital supply source, if asked. Keep in mind that while basic items like soap and tissues may be provided by the hospital, your loved one may appreciate familiar versions of these things from home. Talk to your loved one about what you can do to assist. And always check with her physician or nurse whether the suggestions made in this book are appropriate and acceptable for her before following any of them.

❖ *58.* Bring some mouth swabs and locate the hospital-supplied bedside spit bowl. Swabs can cleanse teeth, tongue, and gums when the mouth area is too sensitive for normal toothbrushing and oral hygiene routines. They are available from hospital supply stores as either disposable foam-rubber–tipped sticks or individually wrapped lemon moistened mouth swabs. A homemade version can be improvised with Q-tips, plain or gauze wrapped.

❖ *59.* Bring a bottle of Salivert, an artificial spray saliva that is effective for ten to thirty minutes, to relieve dry mouth. (Available over the counter in pharmacies.)

❖ 60. Bring a pocket-sized spray mouthwash and some sucking mints to refresh breath and alleviate dry mouth.

❖ 61. Bring and replenish the ice-chip supply to keep at the patient's bedside. The ice helps counter dry mouth. An ice machine is usually located somewhere on each hospital floor. The smaller the chip, the easier it will be for your loved one to manage in her mouth.

❖ 62. Bring some lip balm like Chapstick or a squeeze tube of Vaseline to relieve chapped lips.

❖ 63. Bring a spray bottle for misting the face with water if normal washing at the sink is too difficult. Water will be soothing and refreshing. Various other solutions may be suggested by the physician or nurse to help cleanse other body parts.

❖ 64. Bring her familiar brands of sanitary/hygiene products, soap, deodorant, and toothpaste. Check with the physician or nurse to be certain these products are permissible for your loved one to use.

❖ 65. Bring a container of moist baby wipes for easy cleaning of hands or other body parts without getting out of bed.

❖ 66. Bring a soft towel from home for wiping hands and face.

❖ *67.* Bring a package of lens papers so glasses can be cleaned without getting out of bed.

❖ *68.* Bring a small wicker basket with a tall handle for holding candies or personal items. The handle will make it easier to grasp and retrieve these items while reclining in bed.

❖ *69.* Bring "chuks," "egg crates," or some other form of cushioned bed pads. If the hospital doesn't provide them, try a surgical or hospital supply store. Lying in one place for too long a time can lead to bedsores. These pads are designed to help distribute the semi-mobile or immobile person's weight. This will alleviate some of the discomfort on existing bedsores and can even help prevent them from occurring in the first place.

8

Bring Wearable Comfort

❖ Along with feeling ill, your loved one is not looking his best. Perhaps the changes are temporary and related to being in bed, in hospital attire. Perhaps they are a result of the illness itself. Whatever the causes, any change in one's usual standards of appearance can be distressing. It can be a constant, unpleasant reminder of the illness and its effects. The outward changes may also threaten his sense of who he is deep inside. Whether or not one's vanity was great or small prior to illness, and whatever the degree of change since, appearance is an issue that affects each person. Providing flattering, easy-to-manage articles of clothing can go a long way toward helping your loved one feel better about himself and thus be better able to face the day.

Remember, too, that hospital-issue clothing is designed for convenient medical uses, but is not necessarily the most comfortable of choices. Even if there are practical medical reasons for using hospital gowns, rather than something from home, there may be accessories that you can provide to help the patient look and feel more like himself.

Sometimes familiar clothing is important to have simply because it carries the welcome smell and feel of home with it. That sense of home can then remain with your loved one after you've left the room.

❖ 70. Bring a sleeping mask to shut out light.

❖ 71. Bring several pairs of soft clean socks to wear in bed and warm feet with poor circulation. Slipper socks with treads or rubber soles are especially good on slippery hospital floors. They can accommodate a degree of swelling, depending on size and brand. They are also comfortable to wear and easy to put on and keep on in or out of bed.

❖ 72. Bring some underwear, oversized if his abdominal area is tender or movement is restricted. This simple gesture can go a long way toward restoring dignity in the hospital setting.

❖ 73. Bring a scarf, cap, turban, or hat if your loved one is unable to groom his hair as usual. It will not be easy to keep his hair clean and styled in the hospital. Treatment and illness may affect your loved one's hair as well. Providing something attractive to wear in bed can be especially helpful in maintaining self-esteem.

❖ 74. Bring a favorite robe, sweater, pajamas, or cozy top to wear in bed. Soft, familiar items can be especially comforting for your loved one to wear against his skin.

❖ 75. Bring a favorite pillow, lap blanket, shawl, throw, or quilt from home. Even if your loved one needs to wear the hospital gowns, he can still enjoy something soft and familiar against his skin.

9

Create Comfortable Surroundings

❖ You want your loved one to feel relaxed and soothed and get the rest she needs. If she is awake and alert, you want to surround her with pleasant and interesting things to look at. You want her to experience agreeable aromas, enjoyable sounds, and no disturbing sensations. All this will help to reduce your loved one's stress, and make her feel as happy and comfortable as possible.

But how can you do all this in a hospital? There are sounds encroaching from other patients—conversations, televisions, visitors. There are noises from the medical staff—coming and going, talking, moving equipment, being paged in the halls, and in the rooms. The walls are boring to look at. Even if they are nicely decorated, they are not like home.

You can help create a more pleasing, more relaxing atmosphere. You can do some simple things to counter the

impersonal surroundings of a hospital room. These suggestions will lift the patient's spirits and help her feel more
connected to her life, friends, and family beyond the hospital walls.

❖ 76. Bring a children's tape player. The buttons are
easier to operate than the adult player's.

❖ 77. Bring a set of headphones to block out hospital
sounds. This will allow your loved one to listen to tapes
whenever she desires.

❖ 78. Bring in some music tapes, soothing nonintrusive
nature sounds tapes (waves, wind, birds), intriguing books
on tape, or recorded messages from family, friends, children.

❖ 79. Surround your loved one with photographs of
friends and family, and especially the young children who
cannot visit.

❖ 80. Bring a picture or poster for the wall opposite the
bed so your loved one has something interesting to look at.
Change the pictures often.

❖ 81. Bring a flowering plant instead of cut flowers. It
won't wilt.

❖ 82. Bring a large-numbered, illuminated bedside clock.
It will help orient your loved one and visitors, with or with-

out glasses, day or night. Remember that hospital time does not always feel like real time.

❖ **83.** Bring a wall calendar with clear, large numbers.

❖ **84.** Bring a solid or spray air freshener for the room.

❖ **85.** Bring some potpourri in a decorative bag; it will be easier to transport than a heavy bowl. Or bring an aromatic dried floral arrangement (such as eucalyptus or pine) or a fragrant plant. Even if your loved one's ability to smell has been impaired, keep in mind that a pleasant aroma in the room will encourage friends and the hospital staff to linger, while giving the patient something attractive to look at.

10

Bring Practical Comfort to the Hospital

❖ One of the most difficult side effects of illness for anyone to cope with is the feeling that you are no longer yourself. There is not a set pattern for if and how and when such a feeling can occur. But in general, changes in a person's normal abilities and activities will make most people look at themselves differently. It will be a challenge for you to help your loved one adjust to any limitations illness may create.

Reading and writing are such basic adult activities that we take them for granted. Should the disease process, general weakness, or treatment side effects interfere with your loved one's ability to perform these ordinary, everyday acts, it can be upsetting. Suddenly, roles your loved one had always taken for granted are no longer possible. It can feel as though he doesn't know himself anymore, as though he has lost something vital, lost, even, who he is. This can be most distressing.

You can help lessen these feelings of frustration, loss, or sadness. The following items are seldom packed in a hospital bag upon admission, but can help a bedridden person read and write and conduct his everyday business with greater autonomy. It is a nice way to demonstrate you see the whole person, not just a patient in a bed.

❖ **86.** Bring in some stationery, a notebook, some note cards, and the like, in case your loved one wants to write or dictate correspondence, lists, or thoughts.

❖ **87.** Bring a felt-tip pen; it's easier to write with while reclining.

❖ **88.** Bring a box or large envelope to hold letters, papers, and all the miscellaneous things one accumulates when immobile.

❖ **89.** Bring in a lap desk or a large, thin, hardcover book for a semi-reclining writing surface.

❖ **90.** Bring an oversized button-style or child's calculator because it is easier for weakened hands to operate.

❖ *91.* Bring a clip-on book light for comfortable reading at any hour.

❖ *92.* Bring an easy-to-use bedside lamp; this is gentler on the eyes than hospital overhead lighting.

❖ *93.* Bring a book holder to reduce arm strain while reading books, letters, or other papers.

11

Bring Amusing Comfort

❖ Many people believe mood works in harmony with the body's ability to heal. The laughter you bring with you, your enjoyment of life's amusing incidents, so important for your own well-being, can influence your loved one's mood and reduce stress. Being able to laugh may help her affirm life and maintain her positive attitude. She may feel strengthened by laughter. It can dispel fatigue and boredom. Or she may simply find it a relief to laugh, to defy fear, or pain, or sadness.

This is not to say jokes and comedy are always appropriate. Evaluate your loved one's desire for mirth and the effect this might have on her. Laughter is suggested only for the benefit of your loved one; you should be careful not to use humor for other ends. Be aware of your own motives— are you entertaining your loved one for her benefit or are you forcing her to be entertaining so you and other visitors

can thereby avoid your own possible discomfort with illness?
Be careful not to use amusement to block the patient's need
to express more serious thoughts and painful emotions. Allow both happy and unhappy feelings a place and a means
of expression.

Always approach humor with a sensitivity to your loved
one's energy level, mood, and needs. Used well, levity can
be a great bond between two people. She may feel, in the
right moment, that it is an affirmation of your relationship
together.

❖ *94.* Bring a favorite book from childhood.

❖ *95.* Bring a collection of jokes, riddles, puns, or
cartoons.

❖ *96.* Bring some kids' comic books.

❖ *97.* Bring a collection of short stories or humorous
essays.

❖ *98.* Bring the new hot, gossipy book.

❖ *99.* Bring the tabloids.

❖ *100.* Tell a funny story that happened to you or your
children.

❖ *101.* Bring an audio tape of a favorite comedian.

❖ **102.** Tell the latest jokes you've heard. Make up some jokes together about the hospital routines.

❖ **103.** Bring a goofy gag present.

❖ **104.** Be silly.

❖ **105.** Smile.

12

Send
Comfort from Afar

❖ If you cannot visit as soon as you would like, do not wait for the big visit you plan next week, or the long letter you intend to write soon. If your loved one cannot tolerate visits at present, do not be offended. If you are distressed, or tongue-tied, or too far away, there are still things you can do. Remember that while your hours and days may fly by, they can proceed at a much slower pace in the hospital. Your loved one may be feeling quite alone and appreciate being remembered in small ways. Don't forget that indirect contact may even be preferable at times, depending on the patient's condition.

As in all things when dealing with a sick loved one, take your cues from his mood. Ask first to ascertain his specific needs and desires before sending or bringing things. Ask how he's eating, sleeping, spending his waking hours, what he likes or dislikes about his routine and surroundings. Your knowledge of the person is your best guide. You will recognize discrepancies in his usual interests and his description of his present situation, and that will give you ideas about what might help. For example, an avid reader who feels too weak to read might appreciate a book holder to prop up a book or a cassette player with books on tape.

Once you are clear what your loved one's exact situation is and what he would like, you can do something, even if you are not able to visit in person. If you are unfamiliar with the community or neighborhood in which the hospital is situated, and your own local businesses are unable to arrange delivery, you may have to do a little sleuthing with the yellow pages or the telephone directory service in order to locate sources for things you want to send. Another good resource is the nursing desk on your loved one's hospital floor. The nurse may have a list of local stores or may be personally acquainted with the neighborhood businesses. National department stores, UPS, and the post office will also assist you in extending comfort from afar. Do not think less of these choices; each has its place.

❖ **106.** Arrange for a store, market, delicatessen, bakery, or candy store to deliver, in your place, some of the suggested food items from chapter 6.

❖ **107.** Arrange for a restaurant to deliver prepared foods such as soups, puddings, sherbet, fruit salad, or a family favorite as discussed in chapter 6.

❖ *108.* Arrange for a pharmacy to deliver some of the suggested body-care items described in chapter 7.

❖ *109.* Arrange for a gift shop or stationery store to deliver some of the practical items, such as potpourri, straws, felt pens, and so on, mentioned in chapters 9 and 10.

❖ *110.* Arrange through the nursing station for the hospital's special services to perform some of the body-care routines discussed in chapter 13. If the patient is at home, arrange for local professionals, such as a hairdresser or manicurist, to make a house call.

❖ *111.* Send one-liner postcards often so your loved one can have something from you to hold in his hands.

❖ *112.* Send cards: greeting cards, humorous cards, sentimental cards, occasion celebration cards, holiday cards. Let them speak for you, saying that your loved one is remembered.

❖ *113.* Send recent photographs.

❖ *114.* Send art work from the children in your life.

❖ *115.* Send a calendar decorated with pictures and phrases showing upcoming holidays and special occasions, and recording recent events in your life to keep your loved one informed.

❖ *116.* Record an audio tape yourself and send it.

❖ *117.* Call on the telephone just to say a quick "hello."

PART THREE

Things You Can Do

13

Give Body Comfort

❖ You want to comfort and soothe your loved one. You want to reach beyond the illness to the person you care for. Physical touch is the most personal and immediate way to express your feelings for your loved one. There are many things you can do that you both might enjoy. Let the tone of your relationship prior to your loved one's illness continue to set the tone now.

A person is touched many times by many hands in a hospital. But the care given by loving hands, that carry with them the affection of a special relationship, comforts in a way that no other touch can. Having a familiar person help with routine care can restore some of the dignity that was relinquished when your loved one became a patient. For you, being involved in these seemingly mundane, though intimate, matters can truly be a gesture of love. For your loved one, the warmth and attention will be immeasurable.

But it is not only affection or assistance you are giving. The results themselves will have a positive effect. Your loved one's body has been undergoing changes because of the illness and treatment. The image she had of herself has become vulnerable, if not shaken, by these changes. Helping maintain her personal grooming during this period can boost your loved one's self-esteem. Helping your loved one feel more like herself at a time when so much seems uncertain and unfamiliar is important. The process itself should be soothing and the final results should be emotionally uplifting to your loved one.

Ask the patient what she would most like you to do to help. Be sure to check with the physician or nurse about any medically indicated restrictions. They will probably also be able to direct or assist you in performing many of the care items suggested here. The medical staff can help obtain or give approval to use particular body-care products, or direct you to where in the hospital you might find the appropriate supplies or service people who can assist. Bear in mind that by helping relieve some of the medical staff's workload in these ways, you will free them up to give your loved one more of the other needed attention only they can provide. The following suggestions can be truly comforting experiences shared between two people. Remember to ask your loved one first what she would like done for her.

❖ *118.* Offer to assist with eating and drinking.

❖ *119.* Offer to wash your loved one's face.

❖ **120.** Offer to assist with your loved one's oral hygiene routine.

❖ **121.** Offer to give his face a shave. A cordless electric razor may be the easiest way for you to do this in bed.

❖ **122.** Offer to apply makeup to your loved one's face. Be sure to provide her with makeup remover and some tissues or disposable cleansing pads for later.

❖ **123.** Offer to apply some favorite cologne.

❖ **124.** Offer to shampoo your loved one's hair.

❖ **125.** Offer to brush and style her hair.

❖ **126.** Offer to massage her head or gently stroke her forehead.

❖ **127.** Offer to give your loved one a manicure. Be sure to provide nail polish remover for later use.

❖ **128.** Offer to massage your loved one's hands.

❖ **129.** Hold hands together.

❖ **130.** Offer to shave her legs. A cordless electric shaver is easiest for shaving in bed.

❖ *131.* Offer to give your loved one a pedicure.

❖ *132.* Offer to massage your loved one's feet.

❖ *133.* Offer to assist her in having a sponge or spray bottle bath.

❖ *134.* Offer to apply some lotion to your loved one's skin.

❖ *135.* Offer to rub her back.

❖ *136.* Offer to assist with her physical therapy exercises, as directed by the medical staff.

❖ *137.* Offer to assist your loved one with dressing in fresh clothes from home.

❖ *138.* Offer to assist your loved one with walking to the bathroom, lowering down on the commode, or obtaining a fresh bedpan or urine bottle, as needed.

❖ *139.* Offer to assist or accompany her in venturing out of her bed or the room, as tolerated.

❖ *140.* You can have any gentle physical contact you and your loved one desire.

14

Give Housekeeping Comfort

❖ We all take for granted the ability to move about freely, lifting and holding objects as we move. But when you're involved with someone who is weak or immobilized due to illness and treatment, you begin to take notice of all the thousands of little energy-draining actions that go into just sitting around. If your loved one is unable to perform simple tasks without assistance, you will see and feel the frustration that goes with a loss of such ordinary independence. It can be difficult to have to ask for help to do things that "should" come naturally. After requesting help, your loved one will have to wait and live by others' time schedules, never his own, before the help arrives. Then when it does, he will have to accept another person's way of doing things, rather than his own style. To top it off, your loved one is expected to be grateful, as we all would be, for the time and caring, the help, the special favors. But it can be draining for him to be constantly grateful for the attentions that he now requires, things he was able to perform independently in the past.

Put yourself in your loved one's place. It will make you more sensitive to the many things our bodies do in the course of a normal day if they are fully functioning. That awareness should help guide you in finding ways to assist the patient. Being involved with him will make it easier for you to understand how such dependence can become a source, or symbol, of frustration, anger, and depression. Eliminating some of your loved one's need to ask for help can be a great relief. By offering to assist with some of these things, you can spare him yet another in a long list of such requests.

❖ *141.* Offer to adjust the light by moving the curtains and turning on or off the lamps and overhead fixtures.

❖ *142.* Offer to adjust the temperature by opening or closing windows, turning down or adding more blankets, or adjusting the thermostat where possible.

❖ *143.* Offer to adjust your loved one's posture by using pillows and the bed controls.

❖ *144.* Offer to remove any unwanted food trays from the room, putting aside desired items for nibbling later.

❖ *145.* Offer to consolidate any partially eaten food or candies.

❖ **146.** Offer to straighten up the room, organize the bedside table, or remove any old newspapers.

❖ **147.** Offer to throw out any wilted flowers, freshen up the arrangements, and water the plants.

❖ **148.** Offer to wash out your loved one's hand laundry in the bathroom.

15

Give Practical Comfort in the Hospital

❖ You know and love someone, and now that person is ill and doesn't always feel like herself. She doesn't always have the strength, or even the interest, in keeping up with her paperwork and phone calls and other personal business. And the harder it is to keep on top of those things when she doesn't feel well, the easier it is for your loved one to simply withdraw from everything and everyone. Many people become depressed when they find they cannot do ordinary tasks with their usual ease. Even if the patient's prognosis for complete recovery is excellent, the temporary experience of diminished strength or mobility can adversely affect her self-image and mood.

And what about you? You are part of that greater world beyond the hospital bed. It is right and natural for you to want your loved one to stay interested in people and events out there, including you. You want her to be the person you know and love. You want her to continue to strive toward wellness. Keeping your loved one involved in your life will help give her goals and purpose, distractions and interests beyond herself and the illness. Mental and emotional attachment to other people and things can exert a powerful draw, enhancing the body's innate healing powers.

However, it will not necessarily be easy for your loved one to maintain a sense of control over the basics of everyday life as physical limitations intervene. With less energy, it can be tempting to give up on some tasks, and the relationships and attachments that go along with them. That is where you can help. There are things you can do to counteract your loved one's inevitable sense of a shrinking universe that accompanies being unable to leave the hospital or even get out of bed, and the increased weakness that results from being ill. You can assist your loved one in accomplishing some of the everyday practical matters by which we exert some personal control over our lives and define our relationships.

Your loved one might want help in some, none, or all of these areas. Or perhaps your loved one may only need assistance in the future, in part and periodically. The important idea is to make it possible for your loved one to hold on to her world. Together you can work out ways for the patient to remain vital and involved in her life from her bed.

❖ *149.* Offer to read her mail aloud.

❖ *150.* Offer to take dictation if your loved one wants to correspond, or address and mail any letters for her.

❖ *151.* Offer to organize, keep track of, and/or pay the household bills.

❖ *152.* Offer to assist her in keeping track of hospital insurance paperwork. You can help with calls to the insurance company or hospital accounting office to clear up any questions or concerns.

❖ *153.* Offer to answer the telephone, assist in manually dialing telephone numbers, or making phone calls the patient has not been able to make.

❖ *154.* Offer to go through your loved one's address book or Rolodex to be sure the entries are legible, accurate, and complete. Work with her to clear up any questions. Copy information so there is a back-up of those important entries.

❖ *155.* Offer to set up a telephone tree among friends and relatives to spare your loved one making repetitious phone calls. This is especially helpful the first day or so when someone goes into the hospital and many people need to be informed all at once.

❖ *156.* Offer to help fill out hospital menu forms. If there are questions, offer to call in the hospital dietitian or convey dietary concerns to the doctor or the nurse.

❖ *157.* Offer to read the newspaper or give a synopsis of the day's news events.

16

Give Practical Comfort from Home

❖ You want to make your loved one's hospital stay as comfortable as possible. Resting easy, however, is as much an emotional state as a physical one. Who hasn't spent a sleepless night worrying about work left undone, mounting responsibilities and duties? Your loved one will have those thoughts as well, as he leaves home and enters the hospital. It is natural to worry about one's home and obligations at this time. No matter how much your loved one perceives that the hospitalization is needed, it can be distressing to leave home and relinquish responsibility for that part of one's life. You can ease the patient's adjustment by offering to help care for his home in his absence.

It is not, of course, simply caretaking duties that you address by helping look after your loved one's home. Home, anyone's home, is a familiar, safe haven. By helping out with your loved one's home, you can serve as an emotional link to an important source of security for him.

You should also keep in mind the possibility that your loved one's concerns about leaving home can be masking concerns about his own health, or fears of ultimately being left alone. By addressing the practical care of his home and possessions, you are indirectly reassuring your loved one about his personal fears of abandonment. For many people, the reassurance that you will stand by their place and things sufficiently demonstrates that they too will not be neglected. For others, working out these house-care arrangements can clear the decks so that the other, more basic concerns can be addressed.

What is most important for you to keep in mind is that your loved one should know and feel that his place in the world, literally and figuratively, is being well looked after. Your assistance in this practical area of house care can demonstrate your intention to "be there" for your loved one in other ways as it becomes needed.

❖ *158.* Bring your loved one's mail from home.

❖ *159.* Offer to find or file papers such as bills, letters, insurance forms, addresses, at his home.

❖ *160.* Retrieve the messages from your loved one's home answering machine.

❖ *161.*   Offer to update the message on his home answering machine. An informative message stating when and how to reach your loved one in the hospital, or who to call for information, can save wear and tear on anyone fielding phone calls.

❖ *162.*   Offer to return anything unneeded to his home if the hospital room or closet has become too crowded. Clothes can be exchanged at home for fresh items.

❖ *163.*   Offer to take care of indoor plants and pets.

❖ *164.*   Do basic housekeeping and straightening up so your loved one has a neat, clean home to return to.

❖ *165.*   Offer to coordinate a temporary stop to newspaper and other deliveries.

❖ *166.*   Offer to take care of any routine car maintenance.

❖ *167.*   Offer to take care of yard work and seasonal home maintenance, water and cut the grass, weed the garden, shovel the walk, change the screens or storms, and the like.

PART FOUR

Things You
Can Do Together

17

Share Comfort Activities

❖ You don't want your loved one to be sick and you want your relationship with your loved one to continue. But she is sick and perhaps now you fear everything has changed and is over. Thinking that, you may be uncertain what to say or do when you contemplate visiting your loved one in the hospital.

It's often easy to lose sight of the person behind the illness. Your loved one may be sick, perhaps quite seriously, but your relationship is with the person, not the illness. You want to have the enjoyment of the relationship despite the intrusion of illness. She will want the same thing as you. You are the one who is probably in the best position to ensure the relationship will continue to flourish. You can bring the relationship to her when you visit by continuing to think of and treat your loved one normally.

When you visit in the hospital, remember you are going

"to be with," not only "to see," someone you care for. That simple thought can suggest shared activities and sources of conversation with your loved one. The alternative, of merely going "to see" someone in the hospital, can be stiff and awkward. Let the way you interact while you visit be guided by your relationship with her prior to illness. By sharing things together you keep that relationship alive.

❖ 168. Reminisce about good times you've had together. Catch up on people or work or activities you share together.

❖ 169. Tell jokes or humorous stories to each other.

❖ 170. Ask your loved one for advice.

❖ 171. Laugh together.

❖ 172. Cry together.

❖ 173. Tape record or video tape a conversation with your loved one.

❖ 174. Take a picture of the two of you together.

❖ 175. Make a list of New Year's resolutions together.

❖ 176. Bring your lunch. Have a meal together on the hospital bed.

❖ *177.* Review old photo albums.

❖ *178.* Play cards.

❖ *179.* Do a jigsaw puzzle or a crossword puzzle together.

❖ *180.* Listen to music together.

❖ *181.* Watch something on television together.

❖ *182.* Hold hands together. Hug and kiss your loved one.

18

Help Your Loved One Give Comfort

❖ Your loved one has so much to give—affection, friendship, solace, comfort, advice. Those qualities do not disappear with illness. And there are people he cares for who need and want these gifts, who need to be put at ease, reassured and comforted. There are people he wants to reach out to, to say or do something special for, or to help them cope with their feelings about illness.

But your loved one has limited energy right now. It may be too difficult for him to do all the things that he would like for those he cares for. It may be too draining to reach out to others and say all he wants to. It can be daunting to think of making conversation with each visitor, explaining the same things time after time, when already fatigued himself. Even if your loved one is feeling physically energetic, it can be an unwelcome emotional burden to have to repeatedly help others, even those he loves, overcome their awkwardness with illness or hospital visits.

You can assist your loved one in making others more comfortable with visiting by conveying the care, affection, and warmth he feels to friends and family who are out of reach. And, just as important, by enabling your loved one to express himself in these ways, you are helping him maintain meaningful relationships. You are also demonstrating your respect for the whole person, the person beyond the illness, who may have greater needs than usual at this time, but also has much to give to others.

❖ *183.* Bring in something to nibble on for the patient to offer visitors. It can help break the ice at the beginning of a visit and will allow your loved one to give effortlessly to guests.

❖ *184.* Bring in a pile of magazines with lots of pictures for visitors to leaf through while your loved one dozes or is attended to by the medical staff.

❖ *185.* Bring in the latest news or some interesting magazine or newspaper articles to share. Read them aloud and leave them for others to look at. This can help get a conversation started when someone is at a loss for words.

❖ *186.* Offer to help your loved one prepare a year's worth of birthday cards that can be mailed at the right time.

❖ *187.* Offer to help your loved one prepare his batch of seasonal holiday cards in advance.

❖ *188.* Offer to help your loved one prepare special letters or tapes addressed to select people. These can be delivered now or in the future.

❖ *189.* Ask your loved one what special messages he would like you to convey to particular people. Suggest that he might write notes in his own hand to special people.

❖ *190.* Ask what hopes, wishes, and advice your loved one has for various people in his life. Talking may be less daunting than composing a formal statement. By participating in this dialogue you can act as your loved one's ambassador, should he be unable to express himself directly.

❖ *191.* Offer to call and invite friends and relatives to visit your loved one as he feels ready.

❖ *192.* Offer to contact far-flung friends and relatives and encourage them to speak with or write to your loved one.

19

Help Others Give Comfort

❖ It is not easy to be up close to someone's pain, illness, injuries, or handicaps. Some people will be frightened by the spectacle. Some people will want to avoid contact, making all manner of excuses. For the sake of your loved one, you can help these people overcome their distress enough to maintain some relationship with your loved one.

On the other hand, your loved one may know many people of whom she is fond but does not see on a regular basis. Perhaps these people do not know about your loved one's current status or are unaware of her condition altogether. By informing these people, with your loved one's consent, you give them the opportunity to give comfort too. In so doing, you extend to your loved one the added care and concern these other relationships bring with them.

Of course, at times your loved one may feel so tired, uncomfortable, or unhappy with the situation that most visitors will be unwelcome. During such a period, you can maintain contact (on her behalf) with others in the outside world. Until your loved one feels able to have visitors again you can convey their well wishes, letting them know when they can visit in the future.

Being the liaison between your loved one and the world provides you with additional support as well. You share a community of concern with the people you are contacting on your loved one's behalf. Their involvement can be a source of mutual support for you. Those who come forward to assist and give comfort to your loved one are helping you shoulder the care-taking activities. They share the responsibilities you have taken on, voluntary but real, and that sharing can be a source of comfort to you.

As with all ideas presented in this book, before embarking on any of these suggestions, talk it over with your loved one. Discuss whom she wants to keep informed and what exactly should be said. Always obtain your loved one's consent before discussing her condition with others or inviting someone to visit. What follows are some suggestions on how you might go about enlisting others' participation in giving comfort, with your loved one's permission.

❖ *193.* Offer to keep your mutual friends informed. Set up a telephone tree to relay news among your acquaintances, sparing your loved one the need to repeat the same information about her current condition with each person. That way, she can just enjoy the visits from people you have already updated on her behalf. She can choose to speak about the condition then as much or as little as she likes.

❖ *194.* Offer to record a "patient report" or "message to my friends" instead of the usual "call back later" message on your loved one's home answering machine.

❖ *195.* If appropriate, contact those mutual friends who do not know about the current status of your loved one's condition and indicate they might visit now, with your loved one's consent.

❖ *196.* Notify any community, charity, religious, social, recreational, and professional organizations your loved one has been involved in so their membership can write or send something.

❖ *197.* Offer to schedule visitors (spread out over the day or the week) so your loved one feels cared for, not alternately overwhelmed and abandoned. If visitors are somewhat scheduled, your loved one can more easily change a visit should she feel indisposed.

❖ *198.* Let your reluctant friends discuss their concerns with you in order to allay their fears and help them begin to relate better to your loved one. Answer their questions openly and honestly. Suggest specific things they can do or bring or say to comfort your loved one and themselves.

❖ *199.* Arrange transportation for those who have difficulty traveling to visit. Offer to accompany others (who may be reticent) on a visit to your loved one.

❖ 200. Meet with friends after a visit to share and give mutual support.

PART FIVE

Hospital Care vs. Home Care

20

Help the Medical Staff Give Comfort

❖ You want your loved one to be well looked after at all times, but especially when you are not in the hospital to help out. You can work with the medical staff to help them understand your loved one's needs, strengths, weaknesses, and concerns. It is important, also, to learn from the medical staff's efforts and expertise. They have been through this experience before and have much to teach you. However, because they are going through it simultaneously with many other people, and will go through it with many more after your loved one is no longer there, they may not always be as receptive and responsive as you would wish. Although they are professionals, they are not immune to the stressfulness and demands of the situation. Your insights will help them focus on your loved one more sensitively. Most of all, you want to establish a good relationship with the medical staff because everyone's goal, yours and theirs alike, is the welfare of your loved one. You will be able to utilize their help best if you know what, and how much, you can realistically expect from the medical staff. They, on the other hand, will respond best to your loved one if their efforts are appreciated, implicitly and explicitly, by you, the patient, friends, and family.

❖ *201.* Share your special insights about your loved one with the medical staff. You can help them be more effective. You can pump life into the term "patient."

❖ *202.* Give the medical staff the chocolates you would have liked to bring to your loved one, who probably can't eat such rich food. Thank the medical staff for their help. They can easily get taken for granted amid the rush and worry.

❖ *203.* Assist the medical staff with routine patient care. It will relieve their workload, and speed up care for your loved one, while channeling your energies usefully.

❖ *204.* Assist the medical staff with discharge planning when a return home is anticipated. Talk over with your loved one what her home care needs might be. Convey this information to the medical staff and help coordinate schedules and deliveries for the home care arrangements. You should realize that a good discharge plan depends on someone like yourself participating on the other end. The medical staff will be grateful for your participation.

❖ **205.** Keep the lines of communication open with the medical staff after your loved one is discharged home. Your contact person will identify him or herself. It will probably be either the patient's primary care physician, the admitting physician if there was a specialized reason for the hospitalization, a visiting nurse, a hospital home care department representative, the hospital social worker or nurse/receptionist who made the discharge arrangements, or the nurse in the patient's physician's office. Whoever the main contact person is, your input can help him or her better monitor your loved one's changing needs so the services provided for her can be improved.

21

Give Your Loved One Practical Comfort at Home

❖ Your loved one may be ready to come home and face a lengthy period of convalescence. Although this day has been eagerly awaited, he may be hesitant now that it has arrived. There are a number of things you can do to reassure your loved one that this will be a successful return home. You can start by helping him articulate any misgivings so they can best be addressed.

Your loved one may be concerned that home is not set up conveniently for his needs. Perhaps he is afraid to be too far from the hospital with its emergency facilities. He may feel the need to be very near the doctor in order to feel safe. Perhaps your loved one is afraid he will not have enough pain medication to feel comfortable through the night when at home. While the hospital is an intrusive place, your loved one may worry, by contrast, about being isolated in the seclusion of his home. People often hesitate to drop in on someone's privacy in their home. They may be concerned that visiting will cause the patient more work. In contrast, a hospital invites public intrusion by establishing set visiting hours. And the hospital personnel buzz in and out of rooms at all hours of the day and night.

If your loved one has recently gone through a harrowing medical experience such as a heart attack, cancer surgery, bout of pneumonia, stroke, or other crisis, and is now returning home cured, he may be reluctant initially to leave the site of his rescue. It is not uncommon to fear a recurrence, to remain anxious about illness and not fully believe at first the good news that one will be all right and may return home.

If, on the other hand, a patient is going home because there is essentially nothing else that can be done for him in an acute-care facility, a hospital, to stop the disease process, then it is a different issue, and the medical plan shifts to keeping your loved one comfortable at home. It should be recognized that going home can then represent a letting go of the hope that the hospital staff could overcome any crisis and keep your loved one alive indefinitely. This can be a frightening step to take, emotionally.

No matter the source of your loved one's doubts, these simple gestures can help restore some of his confidence and smooth the way to a more satisfying return home.

❖ **206.** The hospital discharge plan should include ordering convenient hospital equipment for home use and setting up home nursing care if medically indicated. If home attendants are not being used, then friends and family members can devise their own care-giving shifts once the patient is discharged.

❖ 207.   Many people feel a sense of security in being close to their medical team. Write down and review the visiting nurse schedule, doctor appointments, emergency routines, and relevant telephone numbers. Review the procedure for obtaining more medical assistance while at home, whom to call, when to call, what to look out for, and how to handle the situation effectively and confidently should your loved one develop problems or have discomfort. Write relevant instructions, telephone numbers, and names down and keep them near the patient's bedside or by the telephone. Reassure your loved one that he will be well cared for and monitored while at home.

❖ 208.   Bring a large pill organizer box. Medication schedules do, in part, define the day for many ill people, especially when a great many different medications are required at different intervals. An organizer can help make the medication part of self-care clear and manageable. It also gives the patient visible proof that ample medication is available. This will restore for your loved one some sense of control over his body and his daily routine.

❖ 209.   Organize who will visit, and make a chart showing when. Your loved one will be able to look forward to the visits without being overwhelmed by a cluster one day, followed by a long period alone the next. Also, should he feel unwell, the visit can be easily canceled and rescheduled.

❖ **210.** Do the laundry. Frequent linen changes help a bed-ridden person feel fresher, more comfortable. (Hospitals change daily.) Assist with the large increase in towels and bedding that home care requires.

❖ **211.** Buy, rent, borrow, or contrive a hospital-style bed table. It is easier to use and more comfortable than balancing a heavy tray or leaning toward a table next to the bed.

❖ **212.** Use pillows to approximate a semi-reclining position if a movable hospital bed is not available.

❖ **213.** Locate and utilize local groups or agencies that can provide volunteers, support, coping tips and strategies, equipment, in-home counseling, and many other services. (See chapter 31, "Resources for Comfort.")

22

Give the Family Practical Comfort at Home

❖ If you are a friend, when your loved one is discharged from the hospital to her family's care there is still a role for you. The family of your loved one needs you. They have to maintain their lives in addition to caring for your friend. This is a time when you can make a great difference. There are many things you, as a friend, can offer to her immediate family members, even if the family is not well known to you.

The realities of caring for an ill person at home require extra effort in many areas. Ordinary housekeeping chores increase. Meanwhile, the ongoing needs of other family members, especially children, do not diminish; in fact, they often increase. Managing medical routines and equipment, juggling schedules, and keeping friends and relatives informed can all create a potentially crushing load on the family.

Having friends step in to help out the family becomes especially relevant if the illness goes on for a long time. Your contribution can make the difference between a good experience and a stressful experience for all involved. Assisting the family in providing care is an excellent way to give indirect comfort to your friend. The suggestions that follow should be undertaken, of course, with the family's permission. They are designed to help ease the additional burden that such caretaking imposes on any family, no matter the illness, its severity, or duration.

❖ **214.** Offer to relieve the primary caretaker of his or her duties for a few hours. Take over a shift of hands-on care. Encourage the family to take a short break out of the house, away from your friend. They can return a few hours later with renewed energy.

❖ **215.** Offer to shop or run errands for the family. Suggest picking up essential perishables that need frequent replenishing, such as milk, bread, or fruit.

❖ **216.** Offer to cook a meal for the family. Prepare food that can be frozen and reheated, such as casseroles, soups, and stews, or make salads that can be served without additional preparation.

❖ **217.** Offer to help clean the house.

❖ **218.** Offer to do the laundry.

❖ **219.** Offer to keep track of medical insurance paperwork.

❖ **220.** Offer to help out with child care responsibilities, such as driving the car pool, going clothes shopping, making routine doctor visits, and helping out with dinner, bath, and bedtime.

❖ **221.** Give special attention to the children in the family. Talk to them, listen to them, play with them, go on outings with them, and baby-sit for them.

❖ **222.** Offer to walk the dog. Take the cat to the veterinarian. Pick up the pet supplies.

❖ **223.** Offer to set up a telephone tree among your friend's social group. You could serve as the contact person to convey updates of her condition so that the family is not burdened with constantly repeating these reports.

❖ **224.** Offer to be the liaison for the family. You can enlist other friends to volunteer. Set up a visiting schedule of friends who can run errands, or relieve the family members, or help with hands-on patient care, or who simply, but importantly, want to make a social visit with your loved one. Offer to be the coordinator so that family members are not burdened with ornate scheduling logistics.

❖ **225.** Compile a list of community resources, with telephone numbers, for your loved one's family. Include volunteer organizations and the services they offer, and a choice of local stores, restaurants, and businesses that can pick up and deliver goods and services should the family want to use that option. (See chapter 31, "Resources for Comfort," for additional ideas.)

❖ **226.** Offer to keep track of correspondence for your loved one.

❖ **227.** Offer to notify people from a master list in case of your loved one's death.

PART SIX

Contemplating Death

23

Being Comfortable with Dying

❖ If your loved one is actively dying, then you are in a very hard, confusing, and lonely place. No two people are alike. You bring to this difficult experience your own special qualities as you prepare to lose that unique person, your loved one. Whether or not you are acquainted with death, this death is an experience neither one of you has ever gone through in entirely this way before. Together, you will invent fitting responses to the needs that arise.

The one thing that can be said with certainty about death is that there is no right way to go about dying. And likewise, there are no right things for you to say or do at this time. But whatever beliefs you hold about life and death and dying, or what it means and ought to be, there are some approaches that apply to most situations. They are not answers or directions. Rather, they are attitudes meant to help you live more comfortably with the demands of being near someone who is dying. Think of them as guidelines to mold your actions and responses during this difficult time.

These suggestions do not presuppose an acceptance, or even an awareness of dying on the part of your loved one, although that is generally helpful for most people in this culture. These suggestions are for your own benefit. I hope they will help you relate to your loved one as he is approaching death. I hope these thoughts will give you the confidence to be comfortable with death. If you can become comfortable now with the idea of living with your loved one's dying, then the future will be that much easier for you.

❖ **228.** Accept. Accept your loved one, wherever the person is emotionally. Do not try to change or direct his feelings to suit your own expectations and desires.

❖ **229.** Be there. Be with your loved one, bring your feelings into sync with his, as much as you are able. This will help the person feel less alone in this experience of dying. No matter how well prepared he is, in theory, it is still a new, unknown experience. Ultimately your loved one must die without you. Do not leave him first, emotionally, before he has a chance to leave you in reality.

❖ **230.** Listen. Let your loved one talk to you about whatever he wants. Thoughts and feelings should not be taboo or prohibited. Don't close off words. Don't be frightened by them. You might be closing off your loved one in the process.

❖ **231.** Talk. Don't be afraid you will hurt your loved one if you speak your thoughts and feelings out loud. It probably hurts more to feel left out of the life that continues outside the room and will continue after one is dead. Let your loved one participate in your emotional life, even if some of your thoughts are uncomfortable or sad. Don't assume he does not want to be bothered.

❖ **232.** Say it. You don't know how many chances you will have left to say important, and not so important, things. Don't hesitate and create an opportunity for regret later. Your loved one will want to hear that he is important and special. Be reassured that you cannot harm anyone, no matter how frail their health, by speaking, perhaps out of character, of your deep feelings for him.

❖ **233.** Tolerate. Tolerate your loved one's anger without returning it. Tolerate your loved one's fear without succumbing to it. Rage and distress cannot drive death away, nor protect your loved one from the inevitable. Don't let yourself be driven away instead. In tolerance, look past these emotions to the person you love.

❖ **234.** Express. Find a good source to whom you can express your private feelings and fears. This will help you deal with your loved one's feelings more effectively, honestly, and with greater confidence.

❖ *235.* Know. Know that though you will miss your loved one in the future, your loved one, too, will miss knowing you as you grow and change.

❖ *236.* Remember that you are not alone in these powerful feelings of impending loss.

24

Facing Death with Comfort

❖ If you are present during the moment when your loved one dies, you are in a very special and privileged position. It is as unique a moment in our existence as birth. The parents are witnesses, companions, and helpers to the baby's birth. But that first breath of air, of "life," belongs to the baby alone. So too your loved one's death, that final mile along the road of illness, belongs to your loved one alone.

You are still needed though. Your quiet company up until your loved one's death can ease the way. That, after all, is the best anyone can hope to do, to ease another's transition in or out of life. You cannot stop death, or avoid it, or defeat it, or take your loved one's place in it. You can, however, be alongside your loved one when she dies. Your presence is, and always was, the best comfort you can give.

You too are in need of support and comfort during this period. Turn to those you care for in your life and those who care for your loved one. Take strength from your shared concern and the grief you have in common. You may find, however, that not everyone is able to tolerate this close view of dying. Not everyone will be able to be especially supportive of you as you comfort your loved one during this period. There may be people to whom you have felt close, who are distressed by death in general. You will have to weigh how important it is for you and your loved one to assist those people in becoming more comfortable with death, or whether you should turn to others for support at this time. You may find that someone you've known, but not been especially close with, has experienced similar losses. That person may welcome the chance to extend support and advice to you now.

It is possible, however, that there are people you know who have experienced multiple losses over a short period. Such experiences, rather than making them extra-sensitive and responsive during your loved one's dying, may numb or overwhelm these people with the mountain of grief that they already struggle under. This can be true of those who have lost many loved ones to epidemics, such as AIDS, or the devastation of war and other disasters. They may have had too many recent losses in their lives to fully allow themselves to feel the pain of any more loss (and still be able to function). These people might not be able to extend themselves to you or your loved one at this time as much as you would have wished. Do not be disappointed. People who are in a crisis of their own can be helped to stay indirectly involved, if that is all they can tolerate.

It will be a challenge for you to be there for your loved one as she is dying. Even if you are not there beside her at the actual moment of death, which so often comes during the evening or early morning hours, you may have the opportunity to be close during the days or hours leading up to death. Death may appear inevitable or imminent, and that awareness may make it difficult to think of what exactly to say or do. Do nothing at all but be there. Or look to some of the simple suggestions that follow. You will find your own way in this experience.

❖ **237.** Be brave and calm. Be still.

❖ **238.** Sit close. Hold hands.

❖ **239.** Speak of life. Speak of the things you have been grateful for in her life, in your relationship together.

❖ **240.** Speak of death. Speak with acceptance.

❖ **241.** Speak your heart fully. Tell your loved one what you really feel deep down. Do not miss this opportunity.

❖ **242.** Forgive and seek forgiveness for past hurts.

❖ **243.** Ask for your loved one's blessing.

❖ **244.** Say good-bye.

25

Plan Future Comfort

❖ Your loved one does not want to leave this world and those who are cherished. The future, and all the joys and happiness it holds, stretches out before him and is out of his reach. For some people, it can be helpful to envision a time beyond illness, to express wishes about future activities or celebrations. It can be comforting to talk about the hopes and plans that he is not able to fulfill himself, but would want others to continue in his absence. Anticipating the future together can make your loved one feel he has a share in it. Planning for a particular occasion can give your loved one a real say in what will happen in the lives of those he cares about. For many people a special event sometime in the near future, such as a vacation, can become a goal to move toward, to hold on for. Even when the goal itself is not possible for your loved one to achieve, the planning itself can be pleasurable. It can be an important, gratifying experience to help decide and set up what he would do if he weren't so sick or what he hopes you will do in his honor and memory later.

❖ **245.** Plan a vacation.

❖ **246.** Plan a birthday party.

❖ **247.** Plan an anniversary party.

❖ **248.** Plan a graduation party.

❖ **249.** Plan a religious celebration.

❖ **250.** Plan a holiday gathering.

❖ **251.** Plan a menu.

❖ **252.** Plan a shopping trip.

❖ **253.** Plan a gift list.

❖ **254.** Plan a wish list.

❖ **255.** Plan a legacy.

❖ *256.* Plan a funeral.

❖ *257.* Plan a memorial.

❖ *258.* Plan an eulogy.

❖ *259.* Plan an obituary.

❖ *260.* Plan how to be remembered.

26

Give Comfort to Children

❖ Serious illness and possible death are hard things to explain to anyone, especially to children, whatever their age. As adults, we fear we might harm our children by exposing them to information that we ourselves find intimidating. When the ill person is the child's parent or a close relative or friend, the need for us to find a way to talk with the involved child becomes especially pressing. This is infinitely more so when the child is the ill person.

Whether death is a realistic issue or not for the patient, in the minds of children, death will probably be a real fear that they connect to any serious illness, injury, or medically related separation. Adults are sometimes dismayed at children's unflinching directness. At times their self-centeredness astounds as, for example, they wonder how events in your loved one's illness affect them. Their equating of separation, abandonment, death, and sleep can be daunting to disentangle. Always, they will be studying you, trying to read between the lines, measuring your reactions against your words.

How children's concerns are answered by you depends upon their relationship to you and your loved one, the children's ages, and the illness in question. But before a single word is exchanged, your feelings will have set the tone. Sensitivity to some typical childhood concerns will prepare you to help the children in your life deal with these events. Children will express some of the following concerns directly or indirectly:

❖ Will this happen to me?
❖ Is this my fault?
❖ Will it happen to other grownups I know?
❖ Who will take care of me if you become ill?
❖ How did she get sick?
❖ Why did she get sick?
❖ Can she make me sick?
❖ Will she die?
❖ Will I die?
❖ Will you die?
❖ What happens when a person dies?
❖ What happens when a person is buried?
❖ Will it hurt?
❖ What will it feel like?

Unfortunately, there are no perfect answers to fit every situation or every child. An awareness of your own feelings and attitudes about your loved one's illness is your most important resource. When you draw on your own reactions, your responses will have the greatest impact and ring most true to children. If you are also generally comfortable discussing death and illness, and have accurate information about your loved one, you will have all the necessary tools to give real comfort, in the form of information and honest reassurance, to the children in your life.

But how do you begin to talk to a child about illness and death? You begin wherever the child is. Start with a recap of observable facts as the child knows them. For example, if his father is ill you could begin with the acknowledgment that the child might have noticed that "Daddy's been feeling tired and Mommy's been a little sad lately," and build from there. Describe the things the child knows from his own observations and firsthand experience. Allow the child to corroborate your statements and expand on them in his own words. Don't take a deep breath and rush through this painful explanation smoothly and quickly. It may take several attempts on separate occasions before the child is willing or able to pursue the topic. Don't force it. Allow the child time for some protective denial, initially.

While you are talking, and listening to the child's questions and reactions, keep in mind that the job of childhood is to grow and embrace life and understand it. Your goal in discussing this topic with the child is to help him make sense of what is going on in such a way that will help him continue to grow. You will have to match the child's interest and ability levels. Clearly an ill grandparent who lives in your home will be discussed differently than one who lives two thousand miles away. A two-year-old will need a different explanation than a six-year-old, and that will be different from the conversation with a ten-year-old. Above all, answer the child's concerns, not your own, in addressing this topic. What follows are some cautions and perceptions to keep in mind when trying to help children cope with illness and death.

❖ **261.** Assume the child is more aware of what is going on than just what you have explained.

❖ **262.** Assume that boredom and lack of interest mask fears and concerns.

❖ **263.** Assume the child has more thoughts on the subject than you are hearing.

❖ **264.** Listen for the personal concern hidden behind the question.

❖ **265.** Answer all concerns frankly.

❖ **266.** Give concrete facts.

❖ **267.** Reassure realistically.

❖ **268.** Encourage the child to visit or speak on the telephone with your loved one, depending on the previous closeness of the relationship with the child and mutual comfort with the visit.

❖ **269.** Allow the child to speak his or her mind freely and question what is happening.

❖ **270.** Encourage the child to draw pictures, write letters, or send greeting cards to your loved one.

❖ **271.** Help the child make audio tapes for your loved one.

❖ **272.** Give the child a photograph of your loved one so she or he can keep that person with him or her.

❖ **273.** If your loved one is an especially important person in the child's life, create a small portable picture album of the child and your loved one, documenting some highlights of their relationship.

❖ **274.** Do not force or prohibit contact.

❖ **275.** Do not promise impossible things.

❖ **276.** Do not cover up, ignore, or deny the child's feelings and perceptions.

❖ **277.** Do not confuse your thoughts and feelings with those of the child's.

❖ **278.** If the child will not visit, ask him or her to explain why. Help the child express his or her concerns about visiting.

❖ **279.** Utilize the additional help of a child or family support group, a private therapist, or the medical social worker to assist during this period. (See chapter 31, "Resources for Comfort.")

27

Acknowledge Comfort Given

❖ Your loved one is going to die and it is unfair. No one can change the sad reality of your loss. You will forever after be without this person whom you love. No matter how much time you have had together, it is not enough. How can it be, when death is putting an artificial end to your relationship? And worst of all, no one can alter this scene you must play out. Death will separate you.

Perhaps you feel angry and bitter, as if you have been robbed. Or maybe you are sad and depressed. You are likely to feel all these and other emotions as well, although your loved one has not yet died. Such feelings are inevitable. But although they are natural, although you have a right to feel them, they threaten to get in the way of your remaining time with your loved one. You will have time to feel and explore these things more fully in the future. For now, they interrupt the relationship you still have.

It is difficult to maintain a positive outlook in the face of your impending loss. As your loved one draws closer to death you may be tempted to focus on that future loss. Try to focus on whatever positive aspects you can identify within this experience. You do have cause for great unhappiness, but there will also be things to take comfort from. Don't overlook or take for granted your own important contribution to your loved one's welfare in searching for positive images. Take heart in knowing that you and others have made a difference in the care you have given. To make someone's death better is something significant.

Remember that attempting a positive outlook, realistic and appreciative, can make the present more tolerable. The alternative, to dwell on your bitterness and the unfairness of fate, will only rob you of any good time you have left with your loved one and taint your future memories.

❖ 280. Be thankful for the time you have shared with your loved one.

❖ 281. Recognize the efforts friends and family have made to bring comfort to your loved one.

❖ 282. See the caring that has been behind other people's attempts to help, successful or not.

❖ **283.** Feel what others have given you and your loved one during this time.

❖ **284.** Don't lose sight of your own contributions to your loved one's welfare. They have mattered.

❖ **285.** Appreciate this moment together, that you have it.

PART SEVEN

---

*Taking Care
of Yourself*

28

Gather Comfort for Yourself

❖ You are vulnerable right now. You may feel like a tower of strength, but the closer you are to your loved one, the more at risk you are for suffering the ill effects of stress. What are they? Insomnia, becoming accident prone, forgetfulness, over-indulgence, and exhaustion are but a few of the perils of stress. It is important that you are aware of these danger signs. You need to take care of yourself so you can continue to take care of your loved one.

Keeping up your strength comes in many forms. People who are closely involved with a seriously ill person often neglect their own medical care. They often ignore their own medical symptoms, feeling that they should not complain, thinking "it" is nothing compared to their loved one's condition. They may think nothing "bad" can happen to them when something so serious is already happening to their loved one. Or perhaps they feel they do not have the time to attend to "minor" issues like their own symptoms, which they "ought to tough out." Part of taking care of yourself involves looking after your health.

You have needs too. If you are afraid to let your guard down and feel your own distress because you fear you might be overwhelmed by it, then you are putting yourself under even greater pressure. Denying your own need for support will not make you stronger. It can, however, increase your risk for stress-related problems and future emotional anguish. The closer you are to your loved one, the more careful you should be about taking care of yourself and accepting the support of others who care about both of you.

❖ 286. Gather strength from friends, relatives, and acquaintances who share your feelings for your loved one.

❖ 287. Gather strength from the medical staff who have daily contact with your loved one.

❖ 288. Gather strength from people around you who are going through a similar experience with someone in their own lives. Informal contacts in a hospital setting can be informative, supportive, and very rewarding.

❖ 289. Gather strength through self-awareness. Seek professional help to enhance your efforts and sort through the sometimes confusing, powerful, fast-moving feelings and events. Professionally led peer support groups abound where people going through similar experiences can help each other. There are many private counselors and therapists with experience helping people deal with this very situation and the feelings it generates. (See chapter 31, "Resources for Comfort.")

❖ **290.** Gather strength from your beliefs. Find or compose prayers that have special meaning for you. Join with others who can lend you their spiritual strength and support. Take comfort in their presence and caring.

❖ **291.** Gather strength through preparation. Read books and articles on your loved one's illness, treatment, death, and dying. Read accounts about her emotional journey through these experiences. Feelings and reactions will make more sense, be less surprising.

❖ **292.** Gather strength from your own good health. Take especially good care of your physical condition. Do not ignore little symptoms or neglect routine check-ups and medical or dental care. Do not compare your problems with your loved one's. Your first job is to be well, so you can do all the other things you want to do.

❖ **293.** Gather strength by being careful. Do not indulge in risky behavior. Stress and accidents often go hand in hand. Practice safety and moderation. You are experiencing more than enough hurt. You do not want to hurt yourself "by accident," too.

❖ *294.*   Gather strength by releasing tensions productively. Do not direct anger toward yourself. Beware of acting out anger in self-abusive behavior. Channel your energy into something useful.

29

Give Comfort to Yourself

❖ You have given your loved one so much comfort. It is time now to do something for yourself. You want some comforting, too. What is more important, you need some comforting. You feel the impact of his illness deeply. True, you are not the person who is ill. But illness takes its toll on all of us. You deserve some special attention, an extra boost. And even more important, your loved one needs you to do this for yourself because he still needs you. Do not let yourself burn out. Do something special for yourself that you would not ordinarily do. Giving yourself some of the comfort and care you have given your loved one will help restore your capacity to give more in the future.

❖ **295.** Treat yourself. Replenish yourself. Nurture yourself. Reward yourself. Indulge yourself. Love yourself.

❖ **296.** Buy something frivolous just for you, something you have always wanted.

❖ **297.** Get your hair done. Get new makeup. Get new cologne. Get new shoes.

❖ **298.** Wear something new and wonderful. Wear something old and familiar. Wear something soft and cozy.

❖ **299.** See a film. Listen to music. Go to a museum. Sit in the park. Read a book. Sing to yourself. Take some photographs. Feed the birds.

❖ **300.** Do something creative. Cook. Draw. Paint. Build. Sew. Write.

❖ **301.** Make something wholesome. Bake a loaf of bread. Bake a batch of cookies. Make a pot of soup.

❖ **302.** Plant some flowers. Weed the garden. Water the plants.

❖ **303.** Have a cup of coffee or tea. Have a piece of chocolate. Have an ice-cream cone. Have a really good meal.

❖ **304.** Go for a ride. Go for a swim. Go for a walk. Go for a run.

❖ **305.** Take a break. Take a nap. Take the day off. Sleep in.

❖ **306.** Have a massage. Have a steam bath. Take a sauna. Take a bubble bath. Sit in a Jacuzzi. Take a long shower.

❖ **307.** Exercise. Work out the stress. Work up a sweat.

❖ **308.** Meditate. Go to religious services.

❖ **309.** Get together with people who know your loved one and give one another mutual support.

❖ **310.** Get together with people who do not know your loved one and be the center of attention.

❖ **311.** Let someone take care of you. Let the waiter serve you. Let the hairdresser pamper you. Let the store clerk wait on you.

❖ **312.** Visit a friend. Pet a dog. Smell some flowers. Hold a baby.

30

Be Comforted

❖ You feel helpless. You think you failed somehow or did not do enough. It is a universal feeling. Being the healthy one, the one who is not ill, carries its own risks and burdens. You may feel guilty for being luckier. You may feel guilty that you did not suffer, or because you could not take all the suffering away from your loved one. This is all the more true if she dies. Some people feel guilty that they could not protect the person they love from becoming ill to begin with, nor rescue her from death. These are natural but totally unrealistic expectations. Take comfort from the fact that you are making a difference. And though your troubling thoughts are normal, they are neither accurate nor productive. Talk about these and related concerns with friends, clergy, professional counselors, and others who have a loved one who is ill. And always appreciate the importance of your contributions to her comfort. What follows are several thoughts to keep in mind.

❖ **313.** Know that your presence is enough. Tolerate your own inaction. Sometimes your loved one might need you to just be there in companionship, in stillness and silence.

❖ **314.** Know that you are doing all you can do. You will feel better about yourself now, and in the future.

❖ **315.** Know that there is no one right way to go about this.

❖ **316.** Know that you cannot really make this situation all right. No one can.

❖ **317.** Know that you must be extra careful to take good care of yourself during this time.

❖ **318.** Know that your loved one is ill. You are not.

❖ **319.** Know that you are not alone in this experience.

❖ **320.** Know that you are not alone in your feelings.

❖ **321.** Know that this experience has changed you.

❖ *322.* Know that all you do has taught others how to give comfort as well.

❖ *323.* Know that your caring has made this situation better for your loved one.

❖ *324.* Know that without you this situation would have been worse for your loved one.

❖ *325.* Know that all you do has mattered to your loved one.

31

Resources for Comfort

❖ The following telephone clearinghouses, networks, information centers, service centers, and hotlines are all excellent sources for a myriad of illness-related issues. A brief description of each organization's services is provided. Call these numbers without hesitation. These organizations were formed with just such a person as you in mind. Discuss your situation with the trained staff members. They will help you better identify your needs and specify how they or some other organization can best assist you. They all have, or have access to, information and help that you have probably not even thought of, but may well find useful at this time.

❖ **326.** The Department of Social Work in your area hospital should have the most complete up-to-date knowledge of local resources in their files. Ask to speak with the hospital social worker. If that is not possible, ask the social work department for a referral to the appropriate agency or organization, or hospital sponsored group or service.

❖ 327. Ask the primary physician, the assigned nurse, or the head nurse on the floor for referrals, contacts, and helpful suggestions.

❖ 328. The hospice in your area is an excellent resource. (Check your local yellow pages.) Even if your loved one is not formally involved with the hospice, you can request community resource information. The hospice itself may offer support groups and informational groups to the general public as well.

❖ 329. Recommendations from other people going through a similar experience can be timely and accurate. Anyone who has been truly helped will probably be quite glad to share that information with others going through the same ordeal.

❖ 330. Organizations targeting the particular illness your loved one has may be able to provide: information, assistance, grants, care-giving advice, volunteer help, referrals to reliable home health care agencies, counseling or support groups to help your loved one cope with the illness, counseling or support groups to help you cope with any illness-related stress, and counseling or support groups to help you cope with grief and bereavement. Check your local yellow pages and white pages under headings naming the illness.

❖ *331.* Family service agencies located in your community can offer many of the services described above. They are often listed in the telephone directory under the auspices of a major religious group (Catholic, Protestant, or Jewish). Their services are open to all faiths. In the event they do not directly offer the service or help you seek, they are excellent clearinghouses for local resources. They can probably refer you to the appropriate place.

❖ *332.* Ethnic, religious, or social organizations or clubs may offer members volunteer help and informal support.

❖ *333.* An attorney's legal advice can be tailored to your loved one's individual needs in the important areas of living wills, health care proxies, general wills, financial arrangements, and the current regulations in your state on choice in death and dying. An attorney's advice will be precise and up-to-date in an area of law about which many people have vague notions and assumptions but few people know well. Most people have only partial plans, if any, regarding their legal estate and last wishes.

❖ *334.* 1-800-ACS-2345: The American Cancer Society information line. ACS is a private nonprofit organization. This telephone number connects you with its national center for information about many cancer-related services, including treatment options, referrals to local support groups, and sources of financial assistance for illness and treatment-related needs.

❖ *335.* 1-800-4CANCER: The National Cancer Institute's Cancer Information Service is a federally funded organization. This telephone number connects you with the national office that provides personalized answers with trained staff members. Some of the many topics covered include referrals to local organizations, and the latest treatment and clinical trials through the Physician Data Query (PDQ), the national computerized database on state-of-the-art cancer treatment and research; information on cancer prevention, detection, and diagnosis; and numerous publications available by mail. (Spanish-language information telephone specialists are available.)

❖ *336.* 1-800-658-8898: The National Hospice Organization will provide information about a hospice in your community, wherever you are.

❖ *337.* 1-800-366-CCCF: Candlelighters is a clearinghouse of information for parents of children with cancer. It can provide, among other things, free on-line computer searches to locate medical treatments, free brochures on many related topics, and peer support for parents of children with cancer. Its extensive library is open to the public.

❖ *338.* 1-800-882-6227: National Children's Cancer Society is a hotline for childhood bone marrow transplants. All questions regarding medical information, donors, pledges, and financing can be directed here.

❖ *339.* 1-800-342-2437: National HIV and AIDS Hotline is a federally funded resource, part of the Centers for Disease Control. It assists anyone who has a question on the subject. Its numerous services include giving out general educational information, making local referrals for testing and treatment, and providing practical and financial support and access to its database with up-to-the-moment research and treatment.

❖ *340.* 1-800-722-WISH: Make A Wish Foundation is a private nonprofit organization designed solely to ensure that wishes are granted to children in the United States under the age of eighteen who have any form of life-threatening illness. All provisions surrounding the wish are completely taken care of by the Foundation, with no cost to the family.

❖ *341.* 1-708-990-0010: Compassionate Friends is a national self-help support group for bereaved parents and siblings who have experienced the death of a child and/or sibling at any age or from any cause. They provide a quarterly newsletter, brochures, and referrals to a support group in one of their 660 local chapters across the country.

❖ *342.* 1-805-688-1603: Direct Link for the Disabled has an extensive database listing 12,000 local organizations that provide various services for the disabled. Special needs and disabilities resulting from any cause—including, among other things, chronic illness, rare disorders, and accidents—

can be addressed. Callers receive quite extensive individu-
alized research (mailed to them) for any disability-related
need: legal, medical, practical, emotional, financial, and so
on.

❖ *343.* 1-800-55-CHEMO (within N.J. (908) 233-
1103): CHEMOcare is a non-profit, voluntary organization
providing one-to-one support for cancer patients and their
families undergoing treatment. Recipients are matched with
volunteers who have successfully undergone treatment. Visits are made in person in New Jersey and New York City
and by telephone nationwide.

Remember that all of the above organizations exist to
help you with your questions. You yourself do not have to
be ill to avail yourself of their valuable information and
important assistance. Call them. They want to be of service.

The following blank pages have been supplied for you
to add your own listings of additional resources.

Notes

Notes

Notes

Notes

Notes

Notes